EmpowHER:

wellness, hygiene and YOU

Dr. Anjum Shaikh

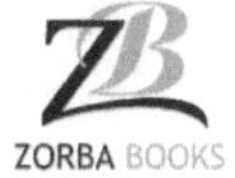

ZORBA BOOKS

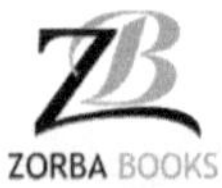

Published by Zorba Books, August 2023
Website: www.zorbabooks.com
Email: info@zorbabooks.com
Author Name: DR. ANJUM SHAIKH
Copyright ©: DR. ANJUM SHAIKH
Title: EmpowHER: wellness, hygiene & YOU

Printbook ISBN: 978-93-5896-716-6
Ebook ISBN: 978-93-5896-717-3

Zorba Books Pvt. Ltd. (opc)
Sushant Arcade,
Next to Courtyard Marriot,
Sushant Lok 1, Gurgaon – 122009, India

Printed in India

"Universal subject of women Hygiene taken care with so much sensually and delicately at the same time it teaches us to celebrate Girl childhood, young lady hood and graceful women hood at the same time and never allowing that girl to grow old! EmpowHER: wellness, hygiene & YOU could be one of the best books for gifting from mother to daughter, at schools and also in the organisations where women folks are working.

Really hope that this book to be multilingual so the reach can be wider and bigger! It handles this universal subject of physical Hygiene, mental Hygiene and spiritual Hygiene in the most beautiful and authentic way! It's so liberating and inclusive.

Anisha Udeshi
Head-Global Insurance & Risk
CIPLA Pvt. ltd

It gives immense pleasure to read a book on woman hygiene & wellness which is a quite unspoken topic because of lots of social taboos. When the information is shared by a young doctor herself "Dr. Anjum Shaikh" this book truly celebrates the journey of womanhood & hygiene.

The celebrations are written in a very witty manner. Some noteworthy special topics touched are menstrual cycle education which gives a good handy information to any young woman who has just achieved her menarche & wants to know more about her journey. Another topic discussed is about eco-friendly products available,which is applauded in protecting the planet earth.

The key element shared in the book is about open communication between partners & health providers. And the final call on menopause is superb with all medically approved information.

There is no doubt that this book will be a great updated source of knowledge to celebrate women-hood & empower women about hygiene & wellness.

Dr. Nilima B Thakur
Consulting Obstetric & Gynecologist
MBBS, DGO, FCPS, DFP

"EmpowHER: wellness, hygiene and YOU!

Indeed, an empowering read for all. A must read for all women, those well informed, partially informed and ignorant. I loved the flow of the content, very relatable and insightful. Takes care of every aspect of well-being and hygiene including emotional wellness, stuff that we need to do proactively, options available and when to start.

What I also loved about the read is a serious subject written in a light hearted manner. You get the inspiration to try it out TODAY.

Mini Nilkund
POSH committee member

EmpowHer is well researched and contains wealth of information in a reader friendly manner from understanding female anatomy, establishing personal hygiene, sexual hygiene, pregnancy and postpartum hygiene to menopause. What sets this book apart is that it also talks about the connection of hygiene to emotional well-being and highlights the significance of self care and self love. The author emphasizes the magic of communication with your partners and with health care providers. Each chapter of the book is covered with actionable tips and guidance for women to take charge of their body and well-being. EmpowHER is all about celebrating women and embracing womanhood.

Shalika Rehani Sharma
Mrs. Bharat USA 2023
Clinical research professional

Dedication

To My Beloved Husband (Dr.Mujib Khan) and Our Precious Six-Month-Old Daughter (Mehr Khan),

With boundless love and profound appreciation, I dedicate this book to both of you, my pillars of strength and my greatest sources of inspiration. As I embarked on the journey of writing this book on female hygiene, your unwavering support and encouragement have been the driving force behind every word penned.

To my husband, you have been my rock, my confidant, and my partner in all endeavors. Your belief in my abilities has given me the courage to pursue this meaningful project. Your endless love has taught me the true essence of empathy and compassion, which reflects in the pages of this book.

And to our darling daughter, though you may be too young to comprehend the significance of this dedication now, I write these words with the hope that one day you will understand the depth of my love for you. As a mother, I am committed to creating a world where you and all women can thrive, protected and empowered by the knowledge within these pages.

Through this book, I aim to raise awareness and break the silence surrounding female hygiene. It is my earnest desire that it serves as a guide for women of all ages, enabling them to embrace their bodies with confidence, understanding, and love.

As I write about the importance of intimate well-being, I am reminded of the importance of nurturing a loving and supportive family. You both are the embodiment of the love and care that every woman deserves. Your presence in my life has given me the strength to pursue my passion for empowering women, including our little one, to grow up in a world where health and dignity go hand in hand.

May this book stand as a testament to the love we share as a family and the values we hold dear. Together, let us continue to uplift and support one another on this beautiful journey of life.

With all my love!

Dr. Anjum Shaikh

Contents

Introduction

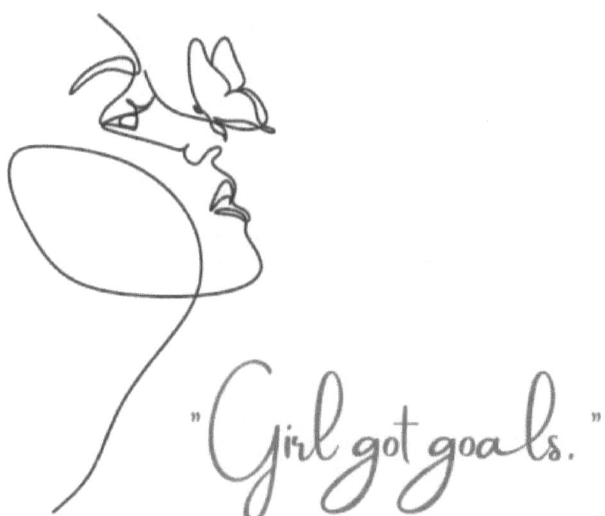

Welcome to "EmpowHER: wellness, hygiene & YOU" This book is a celebration of the beauty and strength of women, offering a comprehensive and empowering exploration of female hygiene and its profound impact on overall well-being. Our aim is to provide you with valuable knowledge, practical guidance, and a sense of empowerment to embrace a healthier and happier lifestyle.

In our journey through these pages, we embark on a voyage of self-discovery and self-care, exploring the wonders of the female body and the intricacies of maintaining excellent hygiene. We understand that female hygiene is more than just a routine; it is a vital aspect of physical and emotional health that deserves careful attention and consideration.

Throughout this book, we encourage an open and positive dialogue about female hygiene, breaking free from taboos and societal norms that have shrouded this essential topic for far too long. We believe in fostering a sense of body positivity and self-awareness, empowering you to embrace your uniqueness and value as a woman.

Our holistic approach covers a range of topics, from understanding female anatomy to embracing menopause and beyond. We delve into menstrual health, intimate well-being, and navigating cultural challenges, all while promoting self-love, self-care, and emotional wellness.

In "EmpowHER: wellness, hygiene & YOU," you will find:

- A comprehensive understanding of female anatomy and the menstrual cycle.
- Guidance on choosing the right menstrual products that suit your individual needs.
- Insights into different feminine hygiene products, including eco-friendly and sustainable alternatives.
- Practical advice for establishing personalized hygiene routines that cater to your unique body.
- Important information on sexual health, safe sex practices, and intimate well-being.
- Tips for navigating pregnancy, postpartum care, and the journey through menopause.
- Strategies to address cultural taboos and embrace positive conversations about female hygiene.
- Encouragement to seek professional advice for optimal health and well-being.

Our hope is that this guide empowers you to embrace your femininity with confidence, compassion, and grace. Let it be a source of knowledge, inspiration, and support as you embark on your journey towards a healthier and happier you.

Remember, you are powerful, you are worthy, and you are deserving of the best care and respect. Together, let's embark on this empowering journey to embrace your true potential and create a life filled with wellness and positivity.

With love and empowerment,

Dr. Anjum Shaikh

Chapter 1

Understanding Female Anatomy

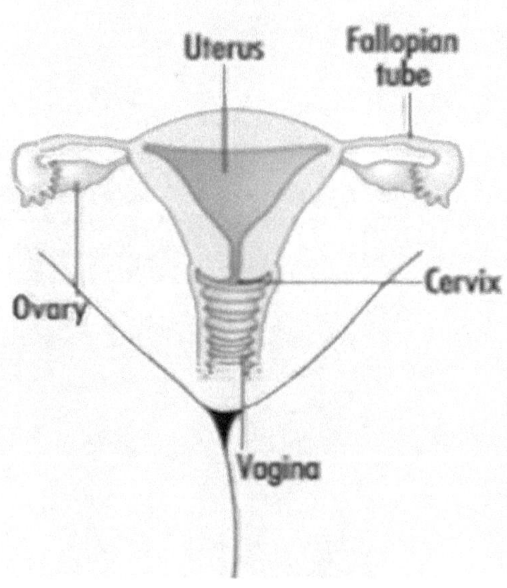

Embarking on the Journey of Womanhood: The Amazing Female Reproductive System

Imagine a world of incredible complexity and wonder that exists within every woman - the female reproductive system. A true marvel of nature, it orchestrates the magic of life and empowers women to embrace their unique ability to bring forth new generations.

Ovaries - _The Seed of Life_: Deep within, nestled on either side of the uterus, lie the ovaries. They are like precious treasure troves, producing and releasing eggs through a process called ovulation. But that's not all! They are also skilled alchemists, crafting essential hormones like estrogen and progesterone, which influence a woman's physical and emotional well-being.

Fallopian Tubes - _A Journey of Hope_: Picture delicate, winding pathways leading from the ovaries to the uterus. These are the fallopian tubes. Every month, like a cosmic adventure, they guide the released egg on a potential quest for fertilization. If an eager sperm meets the egg along the way, a wondrous tale begins - the creation of a new life.

The Uterus - _Nature's Cradle_: Ah, the uterus - a resilient, muscular sanctuary. This incredible chamber is where the seeds of life take root. If the egg becomes fertilized, it settles in the uterine lining, ready to grow into a miraculous bundle of joy during pregnancy. Should the meeting of sperm and egg not occur, the uterus gently sheds its lining, marking the beginning of a new cycle.

The Cervix - *Gateway to Wonders*: At the base of the uterus, lies the cervix, guarding this sanctuary of life. It serves as both protector and guide, releasing special mucus that changes consistency throughout the menstrual cycle, providing just the right environment for conception.

The Vagina - *Gateway to the World*: A gateway between worlds, the vagina connects the cervix to the outside. This versatile canal allows for both the entrance of sperm during fertilization and the exit of menstrual flow. Additionally, it plays a starring role during childbirth, embracing the responsibility of being the birth canal.

The Enchanting External Genitalia: Last but not least, the external genitalia. Like beautifully orchestrated art, they come together to create the labia majora, labia minora, clitoris, and the vestibule. Unique and diverse, they are a testament to the beauty of femininity.

So, dear readers, let's celebrate the wonders of the female reproductive system, an extraordinary symphony of life, and the epitome of womanhood. Remember, taking care of reproductive health through regular check-ups and seeking medical advice when needed ensures this magnificent journey remains enchanting and fulfilling. Embrace the magic of your being, for it's nothing short of a remarkable adventure!

Embarking on an Adventure: Unravelling the Mysteries of the Vagina!

Ladies, let's embark on a journey of discovery as we unravel the amazing world of the vagina! This remarkable part of the female reproductive system has so much to offer, and we're about to dive right in.

1. The Marvellous Vaginal Canal!

Picture this - a flexible and muscular tube that runs like a magical pathway from the outside world to the cervix. We call it the vaginal canal! Not only does it allow for intimate moments with a partner (wink, wink), but it's also the designated exit for menstrual flow during those monthly adventures. And oh boy, during childbirth, it showcases its incredible superpower of stretching like a champ to make way for the little miracles coming into the world!

2. The Mythical Hymen!

Now, let's talk about the hymen - the elusive and often misunderstood little membrane that sometimes says, "Hello, I'm here!" at the vaginal entrance. But guess what? It's not a magic seal of virginity! This little friend can have natural openings or get all stretchy due to everyday activities, so no worries there.

3. The Sensational Bartholin's Glands!

These tiny glands located nearby are like the best-kept secrets of the vaginal world. They're responsible for making sure you have a smooth and delightful ride during intimacy. How? By producing mucus that's your personal lubricant! No friction, only fun!

4. The Enigmatic G-Spot!

Brace yourselves, explorers, for we're about to enter the realm of the legendary G-spot! It's a mysterious spot located on the front wall of the vagina, said to be the gateway to intense pleasure. Not all may find it, but for those who do, it's like uncovering a hidden treasure!

5. The Curious Cervix!

While we're wandering around, let's peek into the cervix's world - the gateway to the uterus. During those romantic moments, it's like a courteous host, pulling back to make room for the excitement. And during menstruation, it opens slightly to let the crimson tide flow.

6. The Elastic Vaginal Rugae!

Our fantastic journey wouldn't be complete without a look at the vaginal rugae. These soft and stretchable folds in the vaginal walls are like acrobats, giving the vagina its elasticity and bounce. They help it bounce back like a trampoline, ready for the next adventure!

So, dear explorers, there you have it - the marvellous and captivating world of the vagina! It's a place of pleasure, wonder, and life itself. Remember, taking care of your reproductive health is essential for a happy and fulfilled journey. If you have any questions or concerns, don't hesitate to seek guidance from healthcare wizards who can sprinkle their magic and keep your adventure smooth sailing! Cheers to embracing the magic of womanhood!

Embrace the Magic of Being a Woman: Celebrating Body Positivity and Self-Awareness!

Hey there, fabulous ladies! Today, we're embarking on a fantastic journey of self-discovery and body love, shining the spotlight on the awe-inspiring wonders of the female anatomy. Get ready to embrace your unique selves and revel in the beauty that makes each of us extraordinary!

1. All Shapes and Sizes are Rockin' It!

Who needs cookie-cutter beauty standards when we've got a dazzling assortment of shapes and sizes? Let's throw out those unrealistic expectations and celebrate the magnificent diversity that makes us true beauties. Whether you're curvy, petite, or somewhere in between - you're a stunning masterpiece, my friend!

2. Every Chapter Tells a Story!

Ladies, our bodies are like captivating novels with numerous chapters! From those first inklings of womanhood in puberty to the incredible tales of motherhood and beyond, our bodies have been through adventures that shaped us into the superheroes we are today! Embrace the journey and wear your life's story with pride.

3. The Marvels of the Menstrual Cycle!

Oh, the magic of the menstrual cycle! It's like a celestial dance of hormones and emotions that make us the fabulous beings we are. Track your cycle, get in sync with your rhythms, and conquer the world like the goddess you are!

4. Fuelling Up with Love and Wholesome Goodness!

Let's ditch the dieting madness and nourish our bodies with love! Fill your plate with delicious, wholesome goodness that fuels your energy and boosts your mood. Remember, self-care is deliciously empowering!

5. Embrace Intimacy and Unleash the Sparks!

Ladies, it's time to celebrate our intimate connections! Our bodies are equipped with sensational pleasure zones like the G-spot, ready to unleash sparks of ecstasy! Embrace your desires and let the sparks fly, because pleasure is your birth right!

6. You are a Unique Gem - Not a Copycat!

No more comparisons, okay? You're an exquisite gem, one-of-a-kind, with your very own sparkle. Say goodbye to imitating others, and hello to celebrating your uniqueness. You are a rare gem in this vast universe, and your light shines bright!

7. Champion of Women's Health!

Knowledge is power, and it's time to claim your crown as a champion of women's health! Educate yourself, prioritize regular check-ups, and support your sisters on their health journeys. Together, we've got this!

8. Love Yourself, Inside and Out!

Ladies, self-love is a superpower! Embrace your imperfections, celebrate your strengths, and shower yourself with kindness. You deserve love, especially from the most important person in your life - YOU!

9. Strut Your Stuff with Confidence!

Confidence is the ultimate accessory! Stand tall, radiate grace, and strut your stuff with confidence. Embrace the magic of self-assuredness, for it's a magnet that attracts all the good vibes!

10. Women Supporting Women - The Ultimate Power Boost!

Let's create a sisterhood of empowerment, lifting each other higher than the stars! Be each other's cheerleaders, celebrate triumphs, and remind one another of our worth. Together, we're an unstoppable force!

Dear fabulous ladies, your bodies are a canvas of endless beauty and strength. Embrace body positivity and self-awareness as you dance to the rhythm of your unique selves. You are powerful, inspiring, and breath-taking - so go out there and conquer the world, one fabulous step at a time!

Chapter 2

Menstrual Health and Hygiene

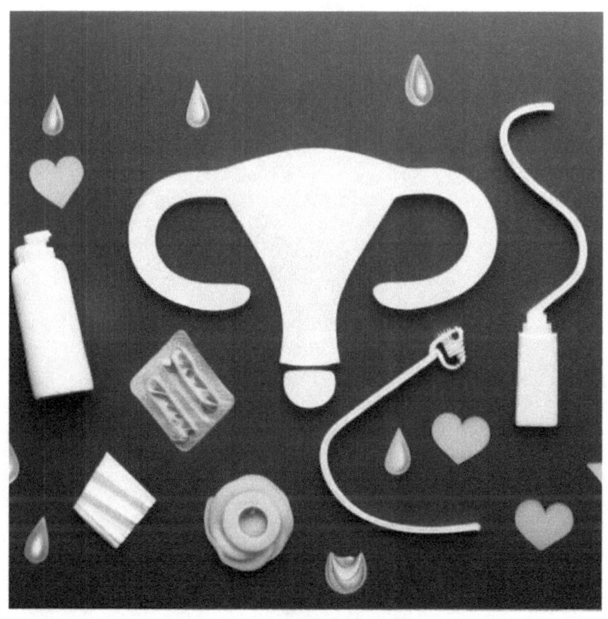

Embrace the Magic of Your Monthly Adventure: Unravelling the Wonders of Menstruation!

Hey, fabulous readers! Today, we're diving into the enchanting world of menstruation - a journey unique to us incredible women. Get ready for an epic adventure filled with knowledge, empowerment, and a dash of sparkle!

1. Unveiling the Marvellous Purpose!

Menstruation, oh what a marvel! It's all about the marvellous preparation for the grand possibility of a new life. When the stage is set, and a lucky egg meets a charming sperm, the spotlight shines bright on the possibility of a little star joining the world!

2. Buckle Up for the Menstrual Cycle Ride!

Ladies, get ready for the roller-coaster ride of the menstrual cycle! It's like a lunar dance of hormones, orchestrating a magnificent symphony of changes in your body. On average, it lasts around 28 days, but hey, don't worry if your cycle has its own rhythm - you're a rock star in your own way!

3. Phase 1: Menstrual Marvels (Days 1-5) - The Big Reveal!

It's showtime! The uterus says, "Lights, camera, action!" as it gracefully sheds its lining - like a curtain call after the previous act. And voilà, the stage is set for the menstrual flow - nature's way of saying, "Hey, we're ready for the next fabulous act!"

4. Phase 2: Follicular Frenzy (Days 6-14) - Egg-tastic Adventures!

Now, it's time for the eggs to strut their stuff! With hormones like estrogen taking the lead, the eggs grow and shine like potential leading stars. They're all hoping for their big break - but only one will take the spotlight!

5. Phase 3: Ovulation Extravaganza (Day 14) - Lights, Camera, Ovulation!

Drumroll, please! The chosen egg, now mature and radiant, steps into the spotlight during ovulation. It's like the perfect casting for a superstar role! This is the golden hour for the egg to meet a charming sperm and create a dazzling new life - a true love story!

6. Phase 4: Luteal Lullaby (Days 15-28) - Cozy Curtain Call!

If the stardust encounter doesn't happen, no worries! The ovary transforms into a superstar producer - the corpus luteum. It pumps out hormones to keep the womb cozy and warm, just in case a pregnancy happens. If not, the curtain falls, and it's time for the next act!

7. Knowledge is Your Superpower!

Knowledge is key, and knowing your menstrual cycle empowers you to conquer the adventure! Keep track of your cycle, listen to your body's cues, and embrace the ebb and flow of each phase. It's like mastering the magic of your body's own secret language!

8. Menstruation - Embrace Your Feminine Power!

Ladies, let's celebrate menstruation as a symbol of our strength and resilience. It's a monthly reminder of the incredible capacity of our bodies and the potential for new beginnings. Embrace this natural process with pride and remember - you're a fierce and fabulous force of nature!

So, dear readers, here's to embracing the magic of menstruation! It's a monthly adventure filled with the wonders of womanhood. Own your sparkle, embrace your rhythm, and know that you're a true superstar!

Finding Your Perfect Match: A Guide to Choosing Menstrual Products!

Hey there, amazing women! When it comes to menstrual products, it's all about finding the one that makes you feel comfortable, confident, and ready to conquer the world during that time of the month. Let's explore the magical world of pads, tampons, and menstrual cups, and discover the perfect match for your individual needs and preferences!

1. Pads - Your Reliable Sidekick!

Pads are like your trusty sidekick, always there when you need them. They come in various sizes and absorbencies, so you can pick the one that suits your flow. They're super easy to use - simply stick them onto your underwear and go about your day with confidence. Pads are perfect for beginners and those who prefer a no-fuss option.

2. Tampons - Freedom to Move!

Tampons are like a ticket to freedom! If you're an active adventurer, they might just be your ideal companion. These little wonder are inserted into the vagina to absorb menstrual flow, leaving you free to move, dance, and jump without worry. They come in different absorbencies too, so you can choose based on your flow and activity level.

3. Menstrual Cups - Eco-Friendly Enchantment

Welcome to the eco-friendly world of menstrual cups! These reusable wonders are like little magic cups that collect your flow. Once inserted, they form a seal and stay put, offering leak-free protection for hours. Menstrual cups are perfect for the environmentally conscious, as they can be used for years with proper care.

4. Choosing Based on Flow and Duration!

Consider your flow and how long your periods typically last. For lighter days, you might prefer pads or liners. On heavier days, tampons or menstrual cups with higher absorbency could be your go-to. Some people even use a combination of products to tailor their protection throughout the cycle.

5. Comfort is Queen!

Comfort is key, ladies! Whether it's pads, tampons, or menstrual cups, make sure you feel comfortable using them. Some may prefer the feeling of pads, while others find tampons or menstrual cups more comfortable. It's all about what feels right for you.

6. Embrace the Learning Curve!

When trying a new product, embrace the learning curve! It might take a cycle or two to get used to using tampons or menstrual cups. Don't worry; practice makes perfect!

Be patient with yourself and don't hesitate to seek advice from friends or online resources.

7. Personal Preferences and Lifestyle!

Your lifestyle and personal preferences play a big role in your choice. Are you a traveler always on the go? Tampons or menstrual cups might be your travel companions. Love the idea of reducing waste? Menstrual cups are a sustainable superstar! The choice is yours!

8. Mix and Match!

Remember, it's okay to mix and match! You can use pads, tampons, or menstrual cups interchangeably based on your activities or preferences. There's no rulebook - only what makes you feel fabulous!

9. Trial and Triumph!

Finding your perfect menstrual product may involve some trial and error, and that's perfectly normal. Celebrate your triumphs along the way, and don't be afraid to explore different options until you find your menstrual soulmate!

10. Listen to Your Body!

Lastly, listen to your body! If a product causes discomfort or irritation, it might not be the right fit for you. Pay attention to how your body responds and make adjustments as needed.

So, dear goddesses, choose your menstrual product with pride! Whether it's pads, tampons, or menstrual cups, the most important thing is that you feel confident, comfortable, and ready to embrace your menstrual magic. Your period doesn't define you, but your choice of product can make it an empowering experience!

Unleash the Magic of Clean and Comfy Periods: Your Ultimate Guide to Menstrual Hygiene!

Hey there, fabulous ladies! Let's sprinkle some pixie dust on your period days and dive into the enchanting world of menstrual hygiene! With a few simple tricks, you'll be ready to rock your period like a true goddess. So, grab your crown and let's discover the wonders of staying fresh and fabulous during your time of the month!

1. Choose Your Period Squad!

Time to assemble your period squad! Pads, tampons, menstrual cups, or period panties - pick the heroes that fit your flow and lifestyle. Embrace your power and remember, each one has its unique magic!

2. Unlock Your Superpower - Clean Hands!

Washing your hands before and after handling menstrual products is like activating your superpower! Zap those pesky germs away and keep yourself protected like the boss you are.

3. Change is the Key to Comfort!

Change is the name of the game, darlings! Swap out your trusted sidekick (pad, tampon, or cup) every 4-6 hours to keep things fresh and fabulous. The more you change, the comfier you'll feel!

4. Keep It Dry and Dreamy!

Let's keep things dry and dreamy, shall we? Swap out that soaked pad or tampon ASAP and opt for breathable fabrics in your undies. Bid adieu to discomfort and say hello to cloud-like comfort!

5. Embrace the Shower Power!

Showers are your secret weapon for feeling fresh and oh-so-fabulous! Take a daily dip and use a gentle, unscented soap to pamper your intimate area. Remember, your vagina is a self-cleaning pro!

6. Bye-Bye Wipes, Hello Love!

Wipes and scented products can't handle your fierce femininity. Embrace the power of love and stick to gentle, unscented products. Your body will thank you with a glowing smile!

7. Rock the Cotton Vibe!

Cotton undies are like your period's BFF - they've got your back! They're soft, breathable, and oh-so-comfy. Bid farewell to irritation and hello to a cottony embrace!

8. Prepare Like a Pro!

You're always prepared for greatness! Toss an extra pad or tampon in your bag, and you'll be ready to conquer the world without a hitch. Period emergencies? Not on your watch!

9. No Toilet-Party for Products!

Remember; don't invite your menstrual products to the toilet-party! Properly dispose of used items in the trash or designated bins. Keep the plumbing happy and the environment smiling!

10. Listen to Your Goddess Body!

Your body is a magical universe, and it speaks to you! If anything feels off, lend an ear, and listen. Reach out to your healthcare provider if you have any concerns - they're your personal guides to well-being!

So, fabulous ladies, with these enchanting menstrual hygiene tips, you're all set to unleash the magic of clean and comfy periods! Embrace your goddess powers and conquer your cycle like the true queen you are. Periods? Piece of cake!

Chapter 3

Feminine Hygiene Products

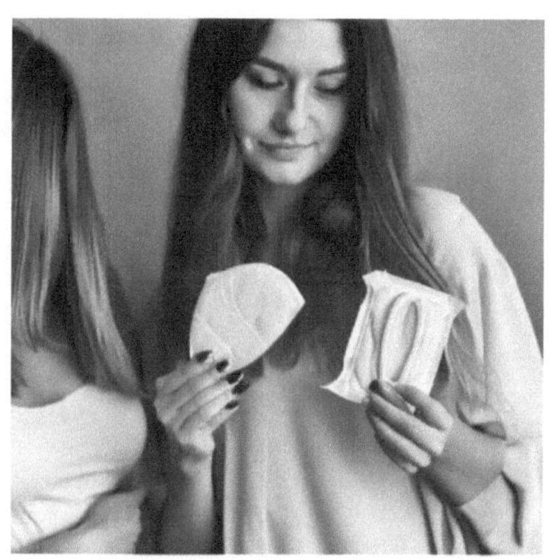

The Magical World of Feminine Hygiene: Unveiling the Pros and Cons of Magical Products!

Hey there, fabulous ladies! Get ready for a mesmerizing journey through the wondrous realm of feminine hygiene products. From enchanting soaps to bewitching wipes and cleansers, each holds its own special powers! Let's uncover the pros and cons of these magical products, so you can make the most dazzling choices for your intimate care needs!

1. Feminine Intimate Soaps: The Gentle Guardians of pH Balance!

Pros: These soaps are like mystical guardians, protecting your intimate area's delicate pH balance. Packed with gentle, natural ingredients, they cleanse without causing a hint of irritation. Some even have soothing powers, perfect for those with extra sensitive skin.

Cons: But beware, not all soaps cast the same spell! Some people might experience irritation due to certain ingredients. Always choose products free from harsh chemicals and artificial fragrances to avoid any unwanted surprises.

2. Feminine Wipes: The Portable Refreshing Spells!

Pros: Feminine wipes are like refreshing spells on the go! With their handy powers, they offer quick and convenient cleansing, making them ideal for freshening up during the day or on magical adventures. Many wipes even carry soothing magic to keep you feeling comfy and confident!

Cons: However, watch out for the wicked ones! Some feminine wipes may contain harsh chemicals or fragrances that could cause irritation. Choose wipes designed specifically for the intimate area to ensure they treat you with the kindness you deserve.

3. Intimate Cleansers: A Mini-Spa Treatment for Your Fairy Garden

Pros: Intimate cleansers are like mini-spa treatments for your fairy garden! They provide thorough cleansing while maintaining a healthy pH balance. Many cleansers come with a no-harsh-chemicals guarantee, so you can indulge in daily use without any worries.

Cons: But like any potion, they might not suit everyone. Some individuals may be sensitive to certain ingredients. Be a cautious sorceress and select cleansers free from dyes, parabens, and sulfates to avoid any spellcasting mishaps!

4. Unscented vs. Scented Products: The Battle of Magical Fragrances

Pros: Unscented products let your natural scent shine through like a radiant star! They're gentle and less likely to cause irritation. Scented products, when chosen wisely, can offer a delightful fragrance to your enchanted routine.

Cons: But beware of the tricksters! Scented products with artificial fragrances may upset your body's natural balance. To avoid any dark spells, stick with unscented options or choose ones with mild, natural scents.

5. The Power of Natural Ingredients: Fairy Godmother Elixirs

Pros: Many feminine hygiene products harness the enchanting power of natural ingredients. With aloe vera, chamomile, and calendula as allies, they can soothe and nourish your intimate area, creating a refreshing and comfortable experience.

Cons: However, every fairy has her quirk! Some individuals may still experience sensitivities to certain natural ingredients. Perform a patch test before regular use to ensure you've got the right potion for your fairy garden.

6. Personal Preferences and Sensitivities: Unleash Your Inner Sorceress!

Pros: Embrace your inner sorceress, for everyone's body is a unique magical realm! Exploring different products allows you to discover the potions that align with your preferences and sensitivities. You hold the power to make empowered choices for your intimate care.

Cons: But remember, the path to finding the perfect potion may involve some trial and error. Don't fret! Each discovery brings you closer to the spellbinding solution.

7. Gentle Care and Embracing Your Body: Unite with Your Magical Essence!

Pros: Gentle care is like uniting with your magical essence! By listening to your body's needs, you empower yourself to make informed choices for your overall well-being. Embrace the enchanting journey of self-care and celebrate your unique body with love!

Cons: There are no real cons to gentle care and self-awareness! The only caution is to choose products free from harsh ingredients that could cause discomfort.

So, dear enchantresses, with this guide to feminine hygiene products, you're equipped to embrace a magical and refreshing experience for your intimate care needs. Choose wisely, stay confident, and remember - you hold the power to make your journey through the enchanted realm a magical one!

Embrace the Natural Magic: Your Ticket to Blissful Comfort!

Hey, gorgeous ladies! Let's embark on an enchanting journey into the world of feminine hygiene products, where nature's magic awaits! Picture this - gentle caresses like a fairy's touch, harmony with your body's essence, and a breath of fresh air in an enchanted meadow. The secret to this wonderland? Choosing natural and chemical-free products! So, let's sprinkle some fairy dust and explore why going natural is the ultimate spell for your happiness and well-being!

1. A Fairy's Tender Caress!

Say hello to the fairy's tender caress! Natural and chemical-free products respect your intimate area's delicate balance, offering you care fit for a magical princess. No harsh additives here - only gentle, soothing ingredients for your comfort!

2. Harmony with Your Body's Symphony!

Embrace harmony with your body's symphony! Synthetic chemicals can cause disruptions and nasty surprises, but natural products keep your magic intact. Say goodbye to irritation and hello to a symphony of blissful comfort!

3. Avoiding Wicked Tricks and Surprises!

Beware of wicked tricks from synthetic ingredients! They promise wonders but may cast spells of irritation on sensitive skin. Choose natural alternatives to steer clear of these mischievous surprises!

4. Like a Breath of Fresh Meadow Air!

Feel the breeze of a fresh meadow! Natural products, filled with the goodness of aloe vera, chamomile, and calendula, offer pure comfort and care. No worries, just blissful moments in the enchanted meadow of your intimate care routine!

5. Eco-Warrior Enchantment!

Calling all eco-warriors! Choosing natural products not only pampers you but also protects our enchanted Earth. Be part of the magic by using biodegradable and eco-friendly options - you're a hero for Mother Earth!

6. Unleash Your Empowered Choice!

Ready to unleash your empowered choice? Embrace your inner enchantress and make conscious decisions for your well-being. Your body deserves the tender magic of nature's care, and you have the power to make it happen!

7. Celebrate Your Unique Radiance!

In this magical realm, every woman is a masterpiece! Natural products celebrate your unique radiance, letting your authentic charm shine through. Embrace your one-of-a-kind beauty - it's what makes you extraordinary!

8. The Sacred Connection to Nature!

Feel the sacred connection to Mother Earth! By choosing natural products, you honor the magic of nature and become part of a bigger enchantment. It's a reminder that we are all connected in this tapestry of wonder.

So, beautiful souls, are you ready for the natural magic? Embrace the beauty of natural and chemical-free products in your intimate care routine, and you'll unlock the gateway to blissful comfort and radiant confidence! Let nature's tender embrace guide you on this captivating journey, and together, we'll create a tale of beauty, empowerment, and joy!

Embrace Eco-Fabulous Feminine Hygiene: Choose Sustainable Options for a Greener Period Journey!

Hey, fabulous eco-warriors! Are you ready to embark on an enchanting journey towards greener, more sustainable periods? Let's explore the magical world of eco-friendly feminine hygiene products that not only pamper you but also show love to our planet. It's time to make a positive impact and create a more sustainable future - all while keeping your period a joyful experience!

1. Eco-Warrior Essentials!

Equip yourself with eco-warrior essentials! Say hello to reusable menstrual cups and period panties. These magical alternatives not only reduce waste but also save you money in the long run. It's a win-win for you and the Earth!

2. Nature's Bounty in Organic Cotton!

Discover the enchantment of organic cotton! Seek out pads and tampons made from this gentle material. They're free from harmful chemicals and pesticides, treating both you and the environment with love and care.

3. Biodegradable Beauty!

Unveil the beauty of biodegradability! Look for products with biodegradable wrappers and packaging. They gracefully vanish back into the Earth, leaving behind no trace of waste.

4. Sustainable Packaging Potion!

Brew the sustainable packaging potion! Opt for brands that use minimal and recyclable packaging. These magical choices reduce plastic waste and ensure your period products are delivered with love to your doorstep.

5. Eco-Friendly Brands that Sparkle!

Support brands that sparkle with eco-friendliness! Look for those committed to sustainability, reducing their carbon footprint, and giving back to the planet. Together, we'll create a world where eco-consciousness shines brightly.

6. Period Cup of Comfort and Freedom!

Unlock the comfort and freedom of a period cup! Reusable menstrual cups offer long-lasting protection and allow you to dance, run, and conquer the world without worries. Plus, they're like a charm for reducing waste.

7. Eco-Enchanted Period Panties!

Step into the world of eco-enchanted period panties! These reusable beauties offer leak-proof protection and are oh-so-comfy. Embrace them like a second skin, as they work their magic to make your period journey greener.

8. Embrace the Power of Reusability!

Embrace the power of reusability! By choosing eco-friendly options, you're reducing the number of single-use products that end up in landfills. It's a transformational spell for a cleaner, happier planet!

9. Celebrate Sustainable Choices!

Celebrate each sustainable choice as a triumph! By choosing eco-friendly feminine hygiene products, you're a beacon of inspiration for others. Together, we'll create a vibrant tapestry of change for a better tomorrow.

10. You're an Eco-Heroine!

Remember, you're not just a heroine - you're an eco-heroine! Every eco-friendly period product you choose contributes to a brighter, more sustainable future. It's time to embrace your magic and change the world, one period at a time!

So, beautiful eco-warriors, let's weave a tale of eco-fabulous feminine hygiene. Embrace the magic of sustainable choices, and together, we'll create a world where our period journey is as enchanting for the Earth as it is for us. Join the eco-fabulous revolution and make your period a greener, more joyful experience!

Chapter 4

Personal Care Routines

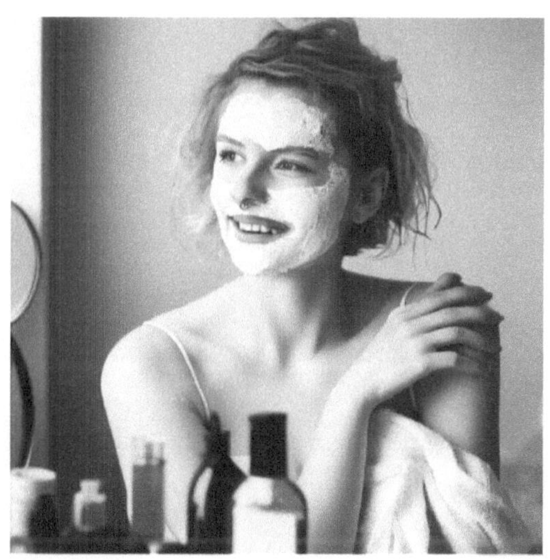

Unleash Your Inner Glow: Craft Your Magical Personal Care Routine!

Hey there, radiant souls! Get ready to embark on a journey of self-love and enchantment as we create a personal care routine that'll leave you shining like a star every day! It's time to weave your magic with these practical tips for your very own personal care wonderland:

1. Listen to Your Body's Whispers!

Your body is your best friend! Listen to its whispers and cues. Pay attention to how it responds to different products and practices, so you can curate a routine that feels tailor-made for your unique magic.

2. Embrace Your Magical Must-Haves!

Discover your magical must-haves! Whether it's a refreshing face mist, a hair serum that tames wild locks, or a body lotion that feels like a hug - let these essentials be the fairy-tale ingredients of your routine.

3. Time It Right for You!

Find the perfect time to sprinkle your self-care magic. Are you a morning sunshine seeker or a night-time moon goddess? Embrace the moment that makes you feel most alive and radiant.

4. Nourish with Nature's Loveliness!

Let Mother Nature be your muse! Seek out products with natural goodness, like a burst of floral extracts or the nourishing embrace of plant-based oils. Mother Nature's treasures are here to pamper you.

5. Create Enchanting Self-Care Moments!

Transform your routine into enchanted self-care moments. Light some scented candles, play your favourite tunes, or immerse yourself in a soothing bubble bath - these are the spells that'll make you feel like royalty.

6. Be an Earthly Enchantress!

Embrace your inner eco-warrior! Opt for eco-friendly and sustainable choices, like reusable cotton pads or products with recyclable packaging. Your care for the planet is part of your radiant glow.

7. Sparkle with Your Personal Touches!

Sprinkle some stardust with personal touches! Make your routine truly yours by adding scents, colors, and textures that delight your senses. This is your canvas to express your magic.

8. Stay Consistently Enchanted!

Consistency is the key to unlocking your magic! Make your personal care routine a cherished ritual - whether it's a daily affair or a weekly pampering session, commit to this enchanted date with yourself.

9. Experiment and Embrace Your Journey!

Let your routine be an adventure, not a rulebook! Try new products or practices to see what makes your heart dance. Embrace the excitement of exploration and celebrate every chapter of your radiant journey.

10. Celebrate Your Inner Glow!

Celebrate YOU in all your magical glory! Your personal care routine is a testament to the love and care you shower upon yourself. Each step is a celebration of the radiant being you truly are.

So, radiant beings, it's time to unlock your inner glow and create your very own personal care wonderland. Embrace the magic of self-love and let your routine be a testament to the enchanting being that you are. Get ready to shine like a star!

Nurture Your Radiant Self: Embracing Daily Care Practices for a Healthy and Happy You!

Hello, beautiful souls! Let's dive into the enchanting world of daily care practices that will leave you feeling refreshed, confident, and in tune with your radiant self. From gentle cleansing to maintaining genital health, we'll explore the magical steps to create a daily care routine that's all about self-love and well-being.

1. The Ritual of Cleansing!

Start your day with the sacred ritual of cleansing. Take a refreshing shower or a soothing bath - let the water cleanse away the remnants of yesterday, leaving you renewed and ready to embrace the day ahead.

2. Embrace Natural and Gentle Products!

Mother Nature's magic is at your fingertips! Choose natural and gentle products for your skin and body. Opt for soaps and cleansers with mild ingredients to pamper your skin with tender care.

3. Radiant Facial Care!

Give your face the royal treatment! Gently cleanse with a facial cleanser suitable for your skin type. Follow up with a moisturizer and sunscreen to shield your skin from the sun's rays and keep your glow intact.

4. Nourish with Moisturizing Magic!

Keeps your skin glowing with moisturizing magic! After cleansing, apply a nourishing lotion or body butter to lock in hydration and leave your skin feeling soft and radiant throughout the day.

5. Enchanting Genital Health!

Embrace the magic of genital health! Wash your intimate area with plain water or a gentle intimate cleanser specifically designed for this delicate area. Remember to avoid harsh chemicals and fragrances that could disrupt its natural balance.

6. A Whimsical Splash of Fragrance!

Sprinkle a whimsical splash of fragrance! If you love a hint of scent, choose a natural perfume or body mist. Just a sprinkle will leave you feeling like a walking garden of enchantment.

7. Cherish Moments of Self-Care!

Throughout the day, cherish moments of self-care. Take a few deep breaths, pause to stretch, or simply gaze at the sky. These little pauses will infuse your day with enchantment and keep you grounded.

8. Stay Hydrated - A Magical Elixir!

Stay hydrated like the enchantress you are! Water is the magical elixir that nourishes your body from within. Keep a water bottle nearby and take sips throughout the day to stay refreshed and energized.

9. The Glow of Beauty Sleep!

Treat yourself to the glow of beauty sleep! Prioritize getting enough rest, as it's the time when your body rejuvenates and renews itself, leaving you even more radiant and ready for tomorrow's adventures.

10. Unleash Your Unique Enchantment!

Remember, you are an enchantress with a unique glow! Tailor your daily care practices to suit your needs and preferences. Embrace the power of self-love, and let your routine be a celebration of your inner beauty and well-being.

So, dear radiant beings, let's weave a daily care routine that's all about nurturing your beautiful self. Embrace these magical practices and make every day a delightful journey of self-love and enchantment!

Unlock the Secrets to Enchanting Feminine Health: An Interactive Journey to Address Vaginal Odor and Balance pH!

Hello, wonderful souls! Let's delve into the enchanting realm of feminine health and explore ways to address vaginal odour while maintaining a healthy pH balance. It's time to nurture your magical essence with care and knowledge for a happy and balanced you!

1. Embrace Your Unique Scent!

First and foremost, embrace your unique scent! Every woman has her own natural fragrance, and it's nothing to be ashamed of. Vaginas have a mild odour that can change throughout the menstrual cycle, which is perfectly normal.

2. Gentle Cleansing with Intimate Care!

Maintain the balance with gentle cleansing! Use plain water or a mild intimate cleanser specifically formulated for your delicate area. Avoid harsh soaps or douches, as they can disrupt your natural pH and lead to odour issues.

3. Breathable, Natural Fabrics!

Let your intimate area breathe with natural fabrics! Choose cotton underwear and breathable clothing to promote airflow, which helps prevent moisture build-up and keeps your pH level in check.

4. Optimal Hydration - Water Magic!

Stay hydrated with the magic of water! Drinking plenty of water helps maintain a healthy pH balance throughout your body, including your intimate area.

5. Avoid Harsh Chemicals!

Be mindful of harsh chemicals! Avoid using scented pads, tampons, or other products with artificial fragrances. These can disturb your vaginal flora and lead to unwanted odour.

6. Probiotics - Friendly Flora!

Consider incorporating probiotics into your diet! These friendly bacteria help maintain a healthy balance in your vaginal flora, supporting your body's natural defences against odour-causing bacteria.

7. Say No to Douching!

Resist the urge to douche! Douching disrupts the natural balance of your vagina, making it more susceptible to infections and odour issues. Your body has its self-cleaning system - let it do its magic!

8. Regular Showers and Freshness!

Prioritize regular showers to stay fresh and clean! After exercise or activities that cause sweating, take a quick shower to wash away any sweat and bacteria that may contribute to odor.

9. Seek Professional Advice!

If you experience persistent or strong odour, consider seeking advice from a healthcare professional. They can help identify any underlying issues and recommend suitable solutions to address the concern.

10. Self-Love and Body Positivity!

Above all, embrace self-love and body positivity! Your body is beautiful and magical, just the way it is. Treat yourself with care and remember that every woman's journey is unique.

So, dear enchanting beings, let's nurture our feminine health with love and knowledge. Embrace these tips to address vaginal odour and maintain a healthy pH balance. Remember, you are beautiful, and your body is a wonderful creation deserving of your care and affection!

Chapter 5

Intimate Health and Sexual Well-being

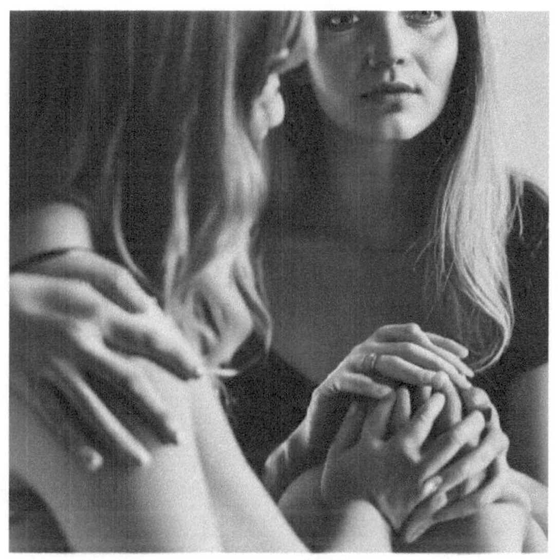

Intimate Health: Embrace the Magical Connection to Overall Sexual Well-Being!

Hello, wonderful beings! Let's embark on an empowering journey to explore the importance of intimate health in nurturing overall sexual well-being. It's time to unlock the secrets to a fulfilling and joyful sexual experience that starts with self-love and care!

1: The Intimate Connection!

Intimate health goes hand in hand with overall sexual well-being. When we prioritize our intimate health, we create a strong foundation for a happy and satisfying sexual life. Let's embrace this beautiful connection!

2: A Journey of Self-Love!

Intimate health is an enchanting journey of self-love. By taking care of our bodies and being in tune with our needs, we embrace our unique beauty and sexuality.

3: Building Trust and Confidence!

Intimate health nurtures trust and confidence in our bodies. When we feel comfortable and in sync with ourselves, we can confidently express our desires and needs in intimate relationships.

4: Enhancing Sensuality!

Intimate health enhances sensuality, allowing us to experience pleasure on a whole new level. By understanding our bodies and desires, we can embrace our sensuality with joy and curiosity.

5: Communication is Key!

Open communication is vital in intimate relationships. By prioritizing intimate health, we can feel more comfortable discussing desires, boundaries, and consent.

6: Exploring Boundaries and Consent!

Respecting boundaries and understanding consent is a magical aspect of intimate health. It creates a safe space for exploration and expression. Let's honor our boundaries and empower ourselves to say "yes" or "no" with confidence.

7: Emotional Well-Being and Connection!

Intimate health extends beyond the physical realm. Our emotional well-being influences our sexual experiences. When we prioritize emotional connection and intimacy, we create deeper and more meaningful connections.

8: Seeking Professional Support!

Sometimes, seeking professional support can be transformative. Whether it's for addressing physical concerns or emotional well-being, remember that reaching out for guidance is a courageous step towards overall sexual well-being.

9: Empowering Your Sexual Well-Being!

You have the power to embrace intimate health and empower your sexual well-being! By valuing yourself, prioritizing self-care, and fostering positive connections, you'll create a harmonious and joyful journey.

So, dear enchanting souls, let's cherish our intimate health and its profound connection to overall sexual well-being. Together, we'll nurture a culture of love, consent, and self-discovery, where every individual's intimate journey is respected and celebrated.

Unveiling the Enchanting Secrets of Sexual Health: Safe Practices and Preventive Measures for STIs!

Hello, beautiful beings! Let's embark on an empowering journey to explore the enchanting world of sexual health, safe sex practices, and preventive measures against sexually transmitted infections (STIs). Together, we'll weave a tapestry of knowledge and empowerment to keep our bodies and hearts safe and thriving.

1: Embracing Sexual Health!

Sexual health is an integral part of our overall well-being. It's about nurturing a positive and respectful relationship with our bodies, embracing consent, and prioritizing our health in intimate experiences.

2: Understanding Safe Sex Practices!

Safe sex practices are like magical shields that protect us and our partners from STIs and unwanted pregnancies. Condoms, dental dams, and regular testing are some of the enchanting tools at our disposal.

3: The Power of Communication!

Open communication is a powerful talisman in intimate relationships. Talking openly about STIs, testing, and contraceptive choices foster trust and enable both partners to make informed decisions together.

4: Regular Testing and Health Check-ups!

Just like a wellness ritual, regular testing is crucial for our sexual health. It allows us to detect STIs early, seek prompt treatment, and protect ourselves and our partners.

5: Stay Informed - Knowledge is Key!

Knowledge is the key to empowerment! Stay informed about STIs, safe sex practices, and contraceptive options. The more you know, the better equipped you are to make informed choices.

6: Prevention against STIs!

Prevention is a powerful enchantment against STIs. Vaccines, such as the HPV vaccine, offer protection against certain infections. Seeking preventive measures and staying informed is a valuable step in safeguarding our health.

7: Avoid Sharing Intimate Items!

Magical items like toothbrushes and sex toys are personal treasures. Avoid sharing them with others to prevent the transmission of STIs. Remember, each enchantress has her unique items!

8: Honouring Self-Care and Well-Being!

Self-care is the ultimate potion for sexual health. By prioritizing our well-being, we can make empowered decisions, embrace pleasure, and foster meaningful connections. How do you prioritize self-care in your intimate journey?

10: Seek Support and Resources!

If you have questions or concerns about sexual health, don't hesitate to seek professional support. Healthcare providers, counsellors, and sexual health organizations are here to empower and guide you.

So, dear enchanting souls, let's weave a world where sexual health is celebrated, consent is honored, and knowledge is freely shared. By embracing safe practices and preventive measures, we'll create a vibrant tapestry of well-being and empowerment. Let's shine brightly in every aspect of our enchanting lives!

Embrace the Magic of Open Communication: Enrich Your Intimate Journey with Partners and Healthcare Providers!

Hello, radiant souls! Let's embark on a wondrous journey of open communication and discover the enchanting power it holds in both our intimate relationships and interactions with healthcare providers. By nurturing this magical skill, we'll unlock a world of understanding, trust, and empowerment.

1: The Art of Sharing!

Open communication begins with the art of sharing. Embrace vulnerability and express your feelings, desires, and concerns with your partner. Sharing thoughts and emotions allows for deeper connections and intimacy.

2: Honouring Each Other's Voices!

Listen with an open heart and honour each other's voices. Create a safe space where both partners feel heard and respected. Embrace differences and celebrate the unique perspectives you both bring to the enchanting table.

3: Embrace Trust and Understanding!

Open communication cultivates trust and understanding. When you feel comfortable sharing your thoughts and experiences, trust flourishes, and intimacy deepens. Encourage your partner to share, knowing that you're there to support each other.

4: Reach Out to Healthcare Providers!

Extend the magic of open communication to your healthcare journey. Feel empowered to share your concerns, ask questions, and seek guidance from healthcare providers. They are there to support and empower you on your path to well-being.

5: Be Curious and Inquisitive!

Curiosity is an enchanting tool! Be inquisitive with your partner and healthcare providers. Ask questions about sexual health, wellness, and preventive measures. The more you know, the more informed decisions you can make.

6: Empowerment through Knowledge!

Knowledge empowers you on your journey. Share information you've learned with your partner and vice versa. Together, you'll create a powerful alliance that values sexual health, consent, and well-being.

7: Embrace Growth and Change!

Embrace the enchantment of growth and change in your intimate relationships and health journey. As you communicate openly, you'll both evolve and grow together, building a strong bond filled with love and acceptance.

8: Seek Support and Guidance!

If challenges arise, don't hesitate to seek support and guidance. Whether through couples counselling or open conversations with healthcare providers, reaching out ensure that your intimate journey is nurturing and joyful.

9: Celebrate Shared Moments!

Celebrate the magical moments of open communication! Whether it's sharing dreams, concerns, or health updates, cherish the bond you create through genuine dialogue with your partner and healthcare providers.

10: Embrace the Power of Love and Care!

Above all, remember that open communication is rooted in love and care. By expressing yourself and listening to your partner and healthcare providers, you'll weave a tapestry of trust, understanding, and well-being.

So, radiant souls, let's embrace the magic of open communication in our intimate relationships and healthcare journey. By fostering understanding, trust, and empowerment, we'll create a world where everyone's voice is valued and celebrated. Let's dance in the enchanting harmony of communication and shine brightly together!

Chapter 6

Pregnancy and Postpartum Hygiene

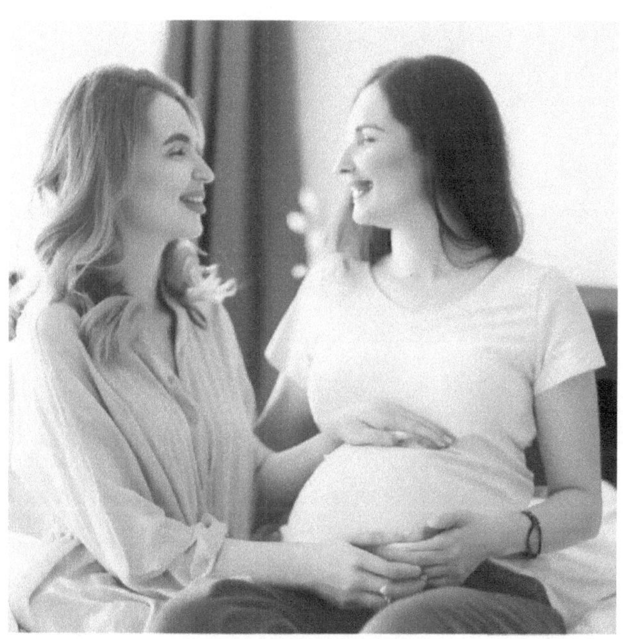

Nurturing the Magic Within: Hygiene Considerations During Pregnancy and Postpartum!

Hello, radiant expectant mothers and new mothers! Let's embark on an enchanting journey to explore specific hygiene considerations during pregnancy and postpartum. Embrace this magical phase with love and self-care as we navigate the wondrous path of motherhood.

1: Gentle and Nourishing Cleansing!

During pregnancy and postpartum, opt for gentle and nourishing cleansing practices. Use mild and natural products for your skin and intimate area. Embrace the beauty of your changing body with tender care.

2: Stay Hydrated - The Nectar of Life!

Water is the nectar of life! Stay hydrated during this transformative phase to support your body's needs. Sip water throughout the day to replenish and nurture your radiant self.

3: Embrace Relaxing Baths!

Treat yourself to relaxing baths! Add natural bath salts or gentle oils to unwind and soothe your body. Bath time is not just for cleanliness but also a nurturing ritual for your well-being.

4: Attend Prenatal and Postpartum Appointments!

Regular prenatal and postpartum check-ups are essential for your health and your baby's well-being. Attend these appointments to ensure everything is progressing beautifully.

5: Embrace Intimate Hygiene!

Take special care of your intimate area during this time. Use unscented and gentle products designed for intimate use. Stay clean and comfortable as your body undergoes its magical journey.

6: Mindful Use of Skincare Products!

Be mindful of skincare products! Choose those with pregnancy-safe ingredients to pamper your skin and prevent irritation. Embrace the glow of motherhood with nurturing care.

7: Prioritize Personal Hygiene!

As you adjust to your new routine as a mother, remember to prioritize personal hygiene. Take showers when possible, and don't hesitate to ask for support from loved ones.

8: Self-Care Moments!

In the whirlwind of motherhood, cherish self-care moments. Whether it's a few minutes of deep breathing or a quick beauty ritual, these moments are precious for your well-being.

9: Seek Support and Guidance!

If you have any concerns or questions about hygiene or well-being, don't hesitate to seek support from healthcare providers or experienced mothers. Sharing experiences can be a powerful source of wisdom.

10: Embrace Your Magic!

Above all, embrace the magic within you! Trust your instincts, be gentle with yourself, and remember that you are an enchanting mother bringing light to the world.

So, dear radiant mothers, let's embrace the enchantment of pregnancy and postpartum with love and self-care. By honouring these specific hygiene considerations, you'll nurture both yourself and your precious little one. May this journey be filled with love, joy, and magical moments!

Embrace the Enchanting Journey: Tips for Cleanliness and Comfort During Pregnancy and Postpartum!

Hello, marvellous mothers-to-be and new mothers! Let's immerse ourselves in an enchanting world of self-care, cleanliness, and comfort during this transformative time. With these magical tips, you'll nurture yourself and your precious little one with love and tender care.

1: Embrace Refreshing Showers!

Take refreshing showers to start your day with a touch of enchantment. A quick shower can uplift your spirits and help you feel clean and rejuvenated.

2: Nourish Your Skin with Gentle Products!

Nourish your skin with gentle and natural products. Choose lotions, oils, and creams with pregnancy-safe ingredients to keep your skin soft and supple.

3: Stay Hydrated - A Magical Elixir!

Stay hydrated like the magical being you are! Sip water throughout the day to support your body and maintain your well-being.

4: Wholesome Nutrition!

Nourish your body with wholesome nutrition. Embrace a balanced diet filled with fresh fruits, vegetables, and protein to support your health and the health of your baby.

5: Intimate Care with Gentle Products!

Take special care of your intimate area with gentle and unscented products. Prioritize comfort and cleanliness during this transformative time.

6: Embrace Sunlit Strolls!

Step into the sunlight for rejuvenating walks. Sunlit strolls can boost your mood and provide a gentle source of exercise.

7: Prioritize Rest and Relaxation!

Listen to your body's whispers and prioritize rest and relaxation. Your well-being is essential for both you and your baby.

8: Embrace Mindfulness!

Embrace mindfulness to stay present in the enchanting moments of pregnancy and motherhood. Practice deep breathing or meditation to find moments of calm and serenity.

9: Comfortable Clothing Choices!

Choose comfortable clothing that embraces your changing body. Embrace maternity wear and loose-fitting garments that allow you to move freely.

10: Seek Support and Share Your Journey!

Surround yourself with a loving support system. Share your experiences with loved ones and seek guidance from experienced mothers who can offer invaluable insights.

So, dear marvellous mothers, embrace these magical tips for cleanliness and comfort during this transformative time. By nurturing yourself, you'll create a beautiful space for the magic of motherhood to flourish. Celebrate this journey, and may each moment be filled with love, joy, and enchantment!

Chapter 7

Menopause and Beyond

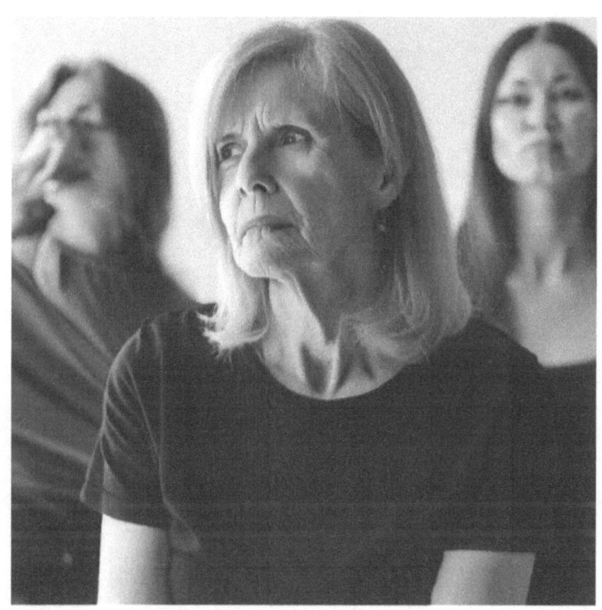

Embracing the Graceful Transition: Hygiene Concerns Related to Menopause and Aging!

Hello, wonderful souls! Let's embark on an enlightening journey to explore hygiene concerns related to menopause and aging with grace and self-love. By understanding and addressing these concerns, we'll continue to shine with radiance and embrace the beauty of every stage of life.

1: Embrace Menopause as a Natural Transition!

Menopause is a natural part of life's enchanting journey. Embrace it as a time of wisdom and transformation. This mind-set sets the foundation for positive self-care during this phase.

2: Prioritize Skin and Body Care!

As our bodies age, tender care becomes essential. Prioritize nourishing skincare and body care routines to keep your skin radiant and hydrated.

3: Stay Hydrated - The Fountain of Youth!

Stay hydrated like a graceful fountain of youth! Water nourishes your body from within and helps maintain your vibrant self.

4: Menopausal Vaginal Health!

Menopause can lead to changes in vaginal health. Stay in tune with your body and consider using a water-based lubricant if needed. Regular pelvic exercises can also support vaginal health.

5: Bone Health and Calcium!

As we age, bone health becomes crucial. Ensure your diet includes calcium-rich foods, and consider supplements if advised by your healthcare provider.

6: Mindful Hair and Scalp Care!

Embrace mindful hair and scalp care as your hair may undergo changes with age. Use nourishing products and consider a haircut that makes you feel fabulous.

7: Regular Dental Check-ups!

Regular dental check-ups are essential for oral health. Maintain a healthy smile and address any concerns promptly.

8: Comfortable and Appropriate Clothing!

Choose comfortable and appropriate clothing that makes you feel confident and radiant. Embrace your unique style while prioritizing comfort.

9: Embrace Gentle Cleansing!

Embrace gentle cleansing practices to maintain your skin's natural balance. Choose skincare products suitable for your changing needs.

10: Embrace Self-Care and Self-Love!

Above all, embrace self-care and self-love during this transformative time. Embrace the wisdom and beauty that comes with aging, and nurture yourself with gentle kindness.

So, dear wonderful souls, let's embrace the grace of menopause and aging with love and self-care. By addressing hygiene concerns with mindfulness, we'll continue to radiate with beauty and wisdom in every chapter of our enchanting lives. Embrace this transformative time, and may each day be filled with self-love, joy, and enchantment!

Embrace the Flow of Change: Adapting Personal Care Routines to Your Ever-Changing Needs!

Hello, radiant souls! Let's embark on an empowering journey to explore ways to adapt our personal care routines gracefully as our needs evolve. By embracing change, we'll create a harmonious self-care dance that celebrates each stage of our enchanting lives.

1: Embrace Self-Reflection!

Start by embracing self-reflection. Regularly check in with yourself to understand how your needs have shifted and what adjustments may be necessary.

2: Mindful Assessment!

Mindfully assess your current personal care routine. Identify elements that still serve you and those that may need modification.

3: Embrace New Priorities!

As your life changes, embrace new priorities. Adjust your personal care routine to align with what matters most to you now.

4: Stay Hydrated - The Fountain of Adaptability!

Staying hydrated supports your body's adaptability. As your needs change, ensure you're nourishing yourself with water's magical elixir.

5: Tailor Exercise to Your Body!

Modify your exercise routine to suit your body's current capabilities and preferences. Listen to your body's whispers and honor its needs.

6: Nourishing Nutrition!

Adapt your dietary choices to support your changing needs. Embrace nourishing foods that energize and uplift you.

7: Addressing Specific Concerns!

As new concerns arise, address them with care. Seek professional advice if needed, and incorporate solutions that promote well-being.

8: Gentle Cleansing and Skincare!

Adapt your cleansing and skincare routines to suit your skin's changing needs. Embrace products that nourish and support your radiant glow.

9: Prioritize Rest and Relaxation!

As life evolves, prioritize rest and relaxation. Ensure you're getting enough sleep to recharge your energy and well-being.

10: Embrace Flexibility and Self-Love!

Above all, embrace flexibility and self-love. Your personal care routine is a reflection of your unique journey, so allow it to adapt and grow with you.

So, dear radiant souls, let's embrace the flow of change and adapt our personal care routines with love and mindfulness. By listening to our bodies and honouring our ever-changing needs, we'll create a harmonious dance of self-care that celebrates each beautiful stage of life. Embrace the magic of adaptation, and may each day be filled with self-love, joy, and enchantment!

Celebrate Your Journey: Embracing Womanhood with Unwavering Confidence!

Hello, amazing women! Today, let's celebrate your journey and empower you to embrace womanhood with unshakable confidence. You are extraordinary, and each phase of your enchanting life is a masterpiece, filled with wisdom and strength. Here are some concrete steps to boost your confidence and revel in the magic of being a woman:

1: Embrace Your Uniqueness!

Embrace the aspects that make you uniquely you! Celebrate your strengths, quirks, and passions, knowing that you bring something special to the world.

2: Embrace Change with Open Arms!

Life is full of changes and growth. Embrace these transformations with curiosity and an open heart, knowing that each experience shapes the strong and resilient woman you are becoming.

3: Embody Strength at Every Step!

Acknowledge your strength and resilience. Reflect on the challenges you've overcome and use them as a reminder of the powerful force within you.

4: Embrace Womanhood with Pride!

Celebrate the diverse expressions of womanhood. Whether you're a mother, sister, friend, or leader, take pride in the roles you play and the impact you have on those around you.

5: Embrace the Journey of Motherhood!

If motherhood is part of your path, embrace it with love and patience. Trust in your instincts and remember that being a nurturing and caring mother is a beautiful journey of growth.

6: Celebrate Your Wisdom and Experience!

Your life experiences have gifted you with wisdom and insight. Celebrate the lessons learned and the knowledge gained as you continue to evolve and inspire others.

7: Embrace New Beginnings Fearlessly!

New chapters bring opportunities for growth and joy. Embrace them with courage, knowing that you have the strength to navigate uncharted territories and create a future filled with endless possibilities.

8: Embrace Self-Expression and Creativity!

Allow your creativity to flourish! Engage in activities that bring you joy, whether it's writing, painting, dancing, or any form of self-expression that fuels your passion.

9: Support and Uplift One Another!

Be a source of support and encouragement to your fellow sisters. Together, we can build a powerful sisterhood that uplifts and celebrates the achievements of every woman.

10: Cultivate Self-Love and Inner Harmony

Treat yourself with kindness and compassion. Prioritize self-care and take time for activities that nourish your soul, whether it's meditating, going for a walk in nature, or simply having a moment of quiet reflection.

So, amazing women, embrace your journey with unshakable confidence. Each phase of life is an opportunity for growth and self-discovery. Celebrate your brilliance, embrace your uniqueness, and let your radiant light shine brightly for all to see!

Chapter 8

Hygiene and Emotional Well-being

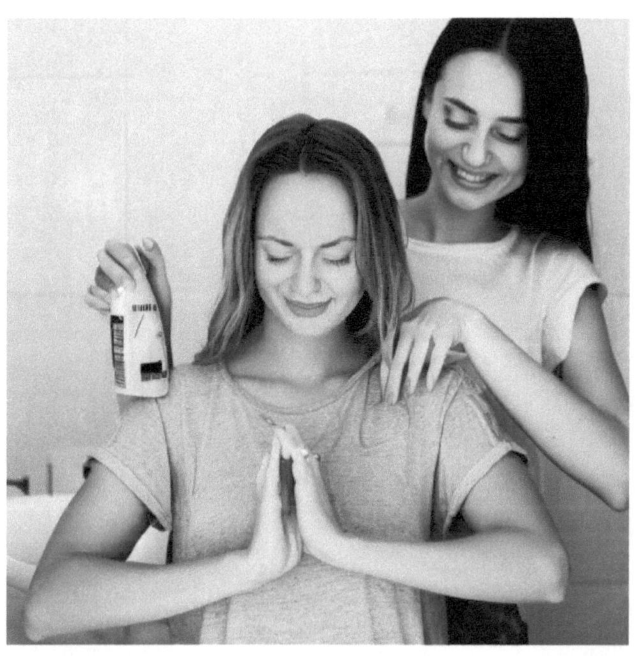

The Empowering Link: Hygiene Practices and Emotional Well-Being

Hello, wonderful souls! Let's explore the powerful connection between hygiene practices and emotional well-being. As we nurture our bodies with loving care, we also tend to our inner world, creating a harmonious dance that elevates our spirits and empowers us to embrace life with confidence and joy.

1: Self-Care as Self-Love

Hygiene practices are an expression of self-love. When we prioritize self-care, we send a powerful message to ourselves that we deserve kindness and respect, fostering a positive relationship with our bodies.

2: The Cleansing Power of Baths and Showers!

Taking relaxing baths or refreshing showers not only cleanses our bodies but also soothes our minds. This sacred time becomes an opportunity to unwind, release stress, and embrace moments of tranquillity.

3: Hydration for Nurturing the Soul!

Drinking water is a nurturing act that keeps us physically and emotionally hydrated. Just like a flower needs water to bloom, our emotions flourish when we prioritize our body's hydration needs.

4: Nutritious Foods for Emotional Nourishment!

Nourishing our bodies with wholesome foods uplifts our emotional well-being. Balanced nutrition supports stable energy levels, positively impacting our moods and overall outlook on life.

5: Embrace Mindful Cleansing Rituals!

Transform daily cleansing rituals into mindful practices. As we wash our faces or brush our teeth, we can also release negative thoughts, allowing room for positivity and self-compassion.

6: Morning Routines for Empowered Days!

Starting the day with a refreshing routine sets the tone for an empowered day. As we groom ourselves, we can set positive intentions, fuelling our emotional well-being for the challenges ahead.

7: Evening Rituals for Tranquil Nights!

Evening hygiene rituals become soothing acts of self-care. As we cleanse and prepare for rest, we let go of daily stresses, creating space for peaceful sleep and emotional rejuvenation.

8: Embrace Sensory Comfort!

Engage your senses in your hygiene practices. Use scents that uplift your mood, textures that bring comfort, and colours that inspire positivity. Allow your senses to nurture your emotional well-being.

9: The Power of Touch!

Through touch, we connect with ourselves. Embrace gentle self-massage or a hug that soothes your soul. The power of touch can nurture emotional healing and strengthen our self-connection.

10: The Confidence Boost of Hygiene!

Practicing good hygiene boosts our confidence and self-esteem. Feeling fresh and clean enhances our self-assurance, making us more comfortable in our own skin and radiating positive energy.

So, wonderful souls, let's celebrate the empowering link between hygiene practices and emotional well-being. As we honour our bodies with tender care, our emotional landscape flourishes with love and positivity. Embrace the magic of self-care, and may your journey be filled with emotional well-being, joy, and the beauty of nurturing your radiant soul!

Self-Care and Self-Love: Essential Elements of Your Healthy Hygiene Routine!

Hello, beautiful souls! Let's embark on a journey of self-care and self-love, recognizing them as vital components of a healthy hygiene routine. By nourishing our bodies and spirits with tender care, we create a harmonious balance that enriches our overall well-being and empowers us to embrace life with grace and joy.

1: Self-Care as a Sacred Act!

Embrace self-care as a sacred act of nurturing yourself. Dedicate time each day to prioritize your well-being, creating a ripple effect of positivity and love in your life.

2: A Love Letter to Your Body!

Treat your body like a treasured canvas. Embrace your unique features and express gratitude for its strength and resilience. Loving your body is the first step towards holistic well-being.

3: Mindful Hygiene Rituals!

Transform everyday hygiene rituals into mindful practices. Embrace the present moment, savouring the sensations and emotions that arise as you care for yourself with tenderness.

4: Nurture Your Mind and Soul!

Your mind and soul deserve gentle care too. Engage in activities that uplift your spirits, such as journaling, meditating, or spending time in nature. Nourishing your inner world is a precious act of self-love.

5: Nourishing Nutrition for Radiant Energy

Treat your body to nourishing foods that support your vitality and well-being. Savor the flavors and take delight in knowing that you are fueling your body with love.

6: Hydration for Inner and Outer Glow

Stay hydrated like the radiant being you are. Drinking water not only nurtures your body but also symbolizes a commitment to self-care and self-love.

7: Embrace Joyful Movement!

Engage in joyful movement that brings you pleasure. Whether it's dancing, yoga, or a refreshing walk, let exercise be an expression of love and care for your body.

8: Soothing Self-Care Rituals

Pamper yourself with soothing self-care rituals. Treat yourself to a relaxing bath, indulge in a face mask, or savour the touch of nourishing lotions. These rituals are acts of self-love that elevate your spirits.

9: Cultivate Compassionate Self-Talk

Speak to yourself with kindness and compassion. Replace self-criticism with loving affirmations. The way you talk to yourself shapes your perception of self-worth and beauty.

10: Embrace Gratitude and Celebrate You

Practice gratitude for the wonderful person you are. Celebrate your achievements, both big and small. Embrace self-love as an unwavering commitment to embracing your radiant essence.

So, beautiful souls, let self-care and self-love be your guiding stars in your healthy hygiene routine. As you nurture your body and soul with tenderness, may you blossom with confidence, joy, and the enchanting beauty of self-love!

Embrace Calmness Within: Promoting Mindfulness and Stress-Reducing Techniques!

Hello, serene souls! Let's embark on a journey of mindfulness and stress reduction, cultivating a peaceful sanctuary within ourselves. By embracing these transformative practices, we'll discover the power to navigate life's challenges with grace and find tranquillity amidst the hustle and bustle.

1: The Art of Mindful Breathing!

Begin your mindfulness journey by tuning into your breath. Take a few moments each day to observe your breath, focusing on its gentle rhythm, and allow yourself to be fully present in the moment.

2: Meditation for Inner Harmony!

Explore the world of meditation, finding a style that resonates with you. Whether it's guided meditation, loving-kindness meditation, or mindfulness meditation, let this practice become your anchor in moments of stress.

3: Relaxation Techniques for Tranquillity!

Discover relaxation techniques that soothe your soul. From progressive muscle relaxation to deep breathing exercises, these tools will help you release tension and embrace serenity.

4: The Healing Power of Nature

Immerse yourself in nature's embrace to reduce stress. Whether it's a walk in the park, a moment by the ocean, or simply gazing at the stars, nature holds the key to calmness and renewal.

5: Mindful Eating for Nourishment!

Turn meals into mindful moments. Savour the flavours and textures of your food, being fully present during each bite. Appreciate the nourishment you provide to your body and soul.

6: Embrace Gratitude and Positivity!

Cultivate an attitude of gratitude, focusing on the positive aspects of your life. Recognize the beauty around you and the many blessings you have, shifting your perspective towards joy.

7: Journaling for Emotional Release!

Give voice to your emotions through journaling. Let your thoughts flow onto paper, releasing any stress and gaining clarity on your feelings.

8: Mindful Movement and Yoga!

Engage in mindful movement, such as yoga or tai chi, to connect your body and mind. These practices promote flexibility and strength while fostering inner peace.

9: Prioritize Rest and Quality Sleep!

Create a restful environment and prioritize quality sleep. Allow your body and mind to rejuvenate, waking up with a refreshed spirit ready to embrace the day.

10: Digital Detox for Mental Space!

Unplug from technology for designated periods to create mental space. Connect with yourself and loved ones without distractions, giving yourself room to breathe.

So, serene souls, let mindfulness and stress-reducing techniques become your compass on this transformative journey. Embrace calmness within, and may these practices empower you to navigate life's waves with grace and find the tranquillity that dwells in your soul.

Chapter 9

Navigating Cultural and Social Challenges

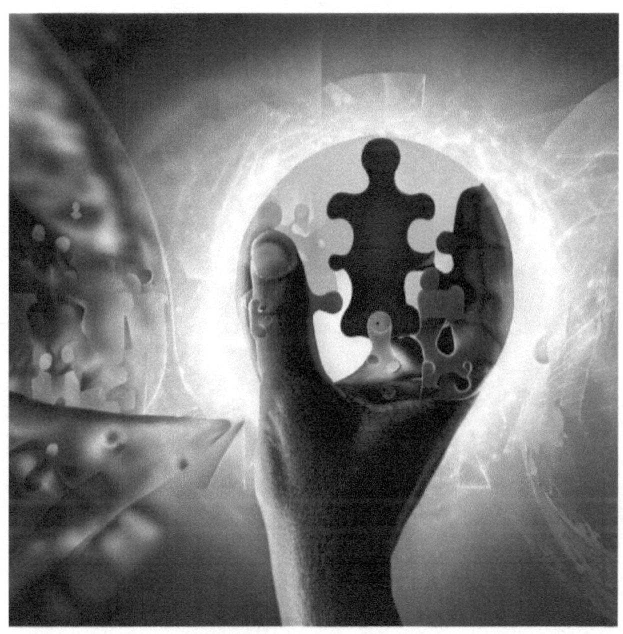

Shattering the Silence: Embrace the Hygiene Revolution!

Hey, trailblazers! It's time to kick down the doors of taboo and dance into a new era of female hygiene empowerment! We're unleashing the power of open conversations and breaking those stifling social stigmas surrounding our hygiene practices. Get ready to join the hygiene revolution and claim our well-being with unapologetic pride!

1: Knowledge is Our Superpower!

Armed with knowledge, we become unstoppable! Get ready to flip the script and learn all about female hygiene with gusto. No more myths, no more shame – we're taking charge of our bodies!

2: Talk the Talk, Break the Taboo!

Girl, let's talk it out! Open conversations are our secret weapon to smash those taboo walls. Gather your squad, your family, or your community and dive into the juicy hygiene discussions like never before!

3: See Ya, Stereotypes!

Sayonara to those pesky stereotypes! We're rewriting the narrative – menstruation is natural, and hygiene is an everyday superhero. No more hiding; we're embracing our bodies with pride!

4: Superhero Advocates for All!

We're donning our capes and becoming advocates for accessible hygiene products. No one should miss out on proper care. Together, we'll fly high and make sure every woman has what she needs!

5: Celebrate Our Cultural Tapestry!

Our beauty lies in our diversity! Let's throw a party of cultural acceptance, celebrating the myriad of rituals and practices around female hygiene. Our unity is our strength!

6: Empowerment Party in Full Swing!

Girls, it's time to rock! Empowerment is our middle name as we lift each other up and build a sisterhood of unstoppable forces. From making choices to smashing barriers – we've got this!

7: Menstrual Talk, No Longer Taboo!

Calling all period warriors! Let's break that menstrual silence and scream it loud and proud. Menstruation is a part of life, and we're here to talk about it without batting an eyelash!

8: Embrace Body Love, Say No to Shaming!

Body shaming, be gone! We're embracing every curve and owning our natural beauty. Our hygiene practices are an act of self-love, and we're flaunting it like a boss!

9: Hygiene Heroes, Unite!

Hygiene heroes of the world, assemble! We're joining forces globally to raise awareness and tackle hygiene challenges. No woman left behind – we've got each other's backs!

10: Solidarity, Our Secret Weapon!

United we stand, unbreakable as one! We're forming communities of support and understanding, sharing experiences and lifting each other up. With solidarity as our superpower, nothing can stop us!

So, trailblazers, gear up for the hygiene revolution! It's time to shake up the world, break down those barriers, and embrace our hygiene journey like never before. Let's roar with pride and claim our well-being with unapologetic zest!

Rise Above Societal Pressures: Let's Empower Positive Hygiene Conversations!

Hey there, amazing souls! Get ready to embark on a journey of empowerment, where we break free from societal pressures and ignite positive conversations about hygiene. It's time to put on your interactive gear and join the revolution! Here's your guide to navigating this exciting path:

1: Be Your Own Cheerleader!

Give yourself a virtual high-five and celebrate your uniqueness! Embrace your personal hygiene choices with pride, knowing that you're rocking it in your own fabulous way. You're a shining star!

2: Let's Talk, Let's Connect!

It's time to unleash the power of conversation! Engage in interactive discussions about hygiene with friends, family, or even online communities. Share your experiences and listen to others' stories. Together, we'll create a supportive platform for positive dialogue.

3: Share Your Hygiene Hacks!

Spread the hygiene wisdom! Share your favourite tips, tricks, and DIY hacks that make your hygiene routine extra special. Let's create a virtual treasure trove of practical and fun ideas to inspire one another.

4: Embrace Your Authenticity!

Break free from the mould and embrace your unique path. Reject societal pressures and unrealistic expectations. Instead, celebrate your authentic self and encourage others to do the same. You're a trailblazer!

5: Celebrate Hygiene Diversity!

Let's throw a hygiene diversity party! Embrace and celebrate the different ways people approach hygiene. Share stories, rituals, and cultural practices that make our hygiene journeys rich and colourful. Every approach is a cause for celebration!

6: Unlock the Power of Fun Facts!

Did you know? Fun facts can spice up hygiene conversations! Discover fascinating titbits about hygiene practices, historical perspectives, or quirky trivia. Share these gems to keep the conversation engaging and entertaining.

7: Create Your Hygiene Mantras!

Words have power! Create personal hygiene mantras that uplift and empower you. Share these mantras with others, encouraging them to develop their own positive affirmations. Together, we'll cultivate a community of self-love and confidence.

8: Virtual High-Five Brigade!

Join the virtual high-five brigade and give kudos to others' hygiene achievements. Celebrate their self-care milestones and encourage them along their journey. Together, we'll build a network of support and positivity!

9: Connect Globally, Inspire Locally!

Expand your horizons and connect with hygiene enthusiasts worldwide. Learn about different cultural perspectives, exchange ideas, and be inspired by diverse hygiene practices. Let's create a global ripple of positive change!

10: Remember, You're an Empowered Hygiene Champion!

You are a superhero in this hygiene revolution! Share your journey, inspire others, and continue to grow as an empowered hygiene champion. Your voice matters, and your positive impact is invaluable!

So, incredible souls, let's rise above societal pressures and ignite positive conversations about hygiene. Together, we'll celebrate our uniqueness, share our stories, and empower one another with interactive and reader-friendly enthusiasm!

Chapter 10

Seeking Professional Help

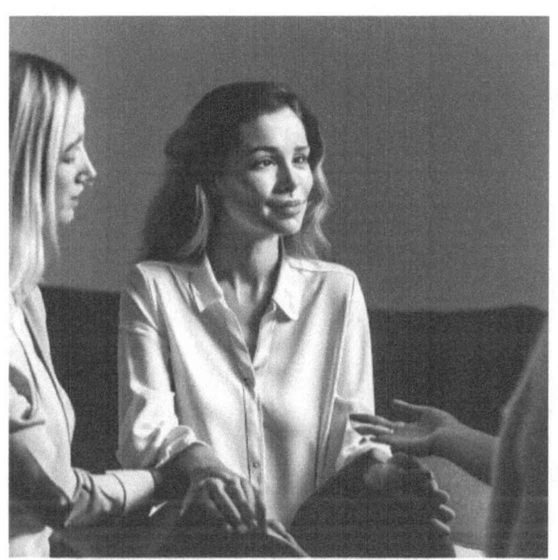

Championing Your Hygiene Health: Rocking Professional Advice like a Superstar!

Hey there, hygiene superheroes! Time to unleash your inner superpowers, and embrace the importance of seeking professional advice for any lingering hygiene concerns. Get ready to rock the stage of self-care and shine like the stars you are! Here's why it's time to take centre stage:

1: Hygiene is Your Superpower!

Your hygiene health is your ultimate superpower! Don't hesitate to reach out to healthcare professionals – they're like your trusty sidekicks, guiding you towards a sparkling hygiene journey.

2: Embrace the Expert Backstage Crew!

Backstage, you've got an expert crew ready to make you shine! Healthcare professionals are your backstage superheroes, providing the knowledge and expertise to tackle any concern.

3: Cue the Timely Intervention!

It's showtime! Don't wait for the grand finale to address concerns. Seek professional advice promptly to put on a dazzling performance of health and well-being.

4: Uncover the Hygiene Mystery!

Get ready to unravel the hygiene mystery! Healthcare professionals are like detectives, finding the clues to identify the root of any concern and providing tailor-made solutions just for you.

5: Hygiene Confidence is Centre Stage!

Confidence is your spotlight! Seeking professional advice boosts your confidence, ensuring you're always ready to shine brightly and rock your hygiene routine.

6: A Health Hero to the Rescue!

Time to call in the health hero! Your healthcare professional is your ultimate ally, standing by your side to listen, understand, and create a strategy to conquer any hygiene challenge.

7: A Show-Stopping Holistic Approach!

Step into the spotlight of holistic care! Your healthcare professional considers your overall well-being, treating you like the superstar you are, and supporting you on every aspect of your health journey.

8: Progress Updates: The Applause of Success!

The applause of success is in your hands! Regular follow-ups with your healthcare professional ensure you're shining brighter with every performance, celebrating your progress like a true star.

9: Expert Recommendations, Your Secret Weapon!

Your secret weapon? Expert recommendations! Healthcare professionals guide you to choose top-notch products, ensuring your hygiene routine is nothing short of award-worthy.

10: Take the Lead: Your Health Journey!

It's time to take the lead on your health journey! Seeking professional advice is like grabbing the microphone and singing your own song of self-care and well-being.

So, hygiene superheroes, let's rock the stage of self-care and champion the importance of seeking professional advice. Embrace the spotlight, embrace your health, and let your hygiene journey be the showstopper of a lifetime!

Unleash Your Health Heroine: Conquering Gynaecological Check-Ups and Nailing Healthcare!

Hey there, health heroines! Get ready to rock the stage of gynaecological check-ups and healthcare like the fierce divas you are! It's time to embrace your health journey with flair and conquer any health challenges with a dazzling smile. Here's your guide to becoming the star of your own health show:

1: Gynaecological Check-Up Extravaganza!

Cue the lights, it's showtime! Your gynaecological check-up is your red carpet moment for reproductive health. Schedule one annually, and let's slay this health game!

2: First-Act Awesomeness!

It's your debut, young women! Your first gynaecological check-up is like stepping into the limelight. Take a bow between ages 13 and 15 or when you become sexually active.

3: The Annual Show-Stopper!

The annual show is a must-watch! For women over 21 or those sexually active, this check-up steals the spotlight, keeping your reproductive health in the spotlight!

4: Selecting Your Star Healthcare Provider!

Casting call for healthcare providers! Choose a gynaecologist or women's health specialist – the stars of reproductive health care. They'll ensure you shine bright with the best care.

5: Curtain Up for Common Concerns!

Common concerns take the stage! If you spot any changes in your menstrual cycle, vaginal discharge, pelvic pain, or any mysterious symptoms, call for an encore with your healthcare provider.

6: Cervical Health: The Cynosure of the Show!

The spotlight's on cervical health! Pap smears are the dazzling routine. From ages 21 to 29, they star every three years. From ages 30 to 65, it's a double act with HPV testing, shining every five years.

7: A Special Act for Special Circumstances!

Special acts, no problem! If you're pregnant, planning to conceive, or have specific health conditions, your healthcare provider will script a personalized show just for you.

8: Trust Your Showstopping Instincts!

You're the director of your health journey! If you feel something's not right or have questions, follow your instincts and call for an encore with your healthcare provider. They're always ready to take the stage.

9: Applause for Your Health Investment!

You're investing in yourself! Let's give a standing ovation for prioritizing your health – it's the star of the show, and you deserve all the love and care!

10: Celebrate Your Health Heroine Journey!

Bravo! Your health journey is a masterpiece. Each step you take is a triumph of well-being and self-care. Celebrate your health heroine journey and keep shining like the dazzling star you are!

So, health heroines, it's time to conquer gynaecological check-ups and healthcare with flair! Embrace your health journey, dazzle the stage with gynaecological check-ups, and remember – you're the star of this health show!

The Grand Finale: Your Spectacular Health Adventure!

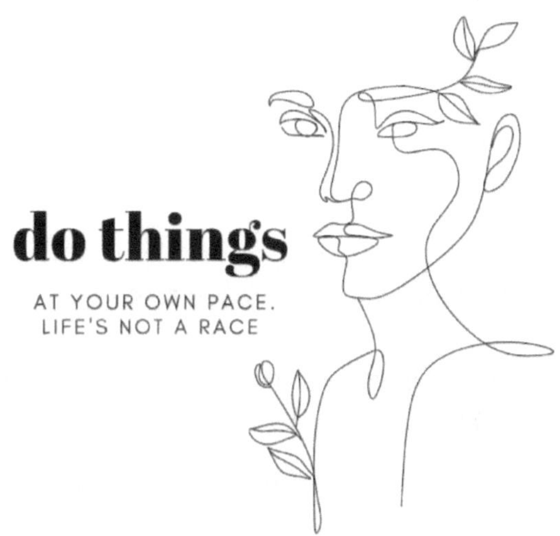

Incredible souls, welcome to the grand finale of your health adventure – a journey that has left us all in awe of your empowerment and self-discovery! From the first act to the last, you've mesmerized us with your enthusiasm and passion for embracing every aspect of female hygiene.

In chapter 1, you fearlessly challenged societal taboos, setting the stage for body positivity and self-awareness. Your charisma drew us in, making us believe that loving ourselves is the greatest show of strength.

Chapter 2 saw you shine brightly, educating us about menstruation and the menstrual cycle. Your knowledge illuminated our minds, turning even the most complicated topics into a fascinating and fun experience.

As you moved on to chapter 3, eco-friendly products took the spotlight, and you transformed the stage into a dazzling showcase of sustainable choices. The applause was thunderous as you proved that protecting the planet can be both chic and responsible.

In chapter 4, your personalized hygiene routine became a masterpiece, a colourful symphony of self-care tailored to each unique soul. We couldn't help but dance along as you showed us that there's no one-size-fits-all approach to health.

Chapter 5 was a journey of intimate health and sexual well-being, and you handled it with grace and sophistication. Your candid discussions reminded us that open communication is the key to building strong and healthy relationships.

With chapter 6, you donned the cape of a superhero, promoting safe sex practices and preventive measures against sexually transmitted infections. Your vigilance was inspiring, and we felt safer just by being in your presence.

Chapter 7 was a heart-warming tale of open communication with partners and healthcare providers. The connection you shared with them was evident, and we couldn't help but admire the trust and support you fostered.

In chapter 8, you embraced the transformative phases of pregnancy and postpartum with tenderness and wisdom. Your nurturing spirit touched our hearts, reminding us of the miracles of life.

As the curtain rose for chapter 9, you gracefully stepped into the spotlight, shining like a diamond in the beauty of menopause and aging. Your resilience and acceptance left us in awe of your strength.

And now, in this spectacular finale, you taught us the importance of mindfulness and stress-reducing techniques. You showed us that the art of self-care is a performance that nourishes the soul and uplifts the spirit.

As the final applause echoes through the auditorium, remember that your health adventure doesn't end here. This is just the beginning of a lifetime of self-empowerment, love, and celebration.

You are the stars of your own show, the heroes and heroines of your unique health journey. And as you continue to shine, may your empowerment inspire others to embrace their own health odyssey with the same zest and passion.

So, let's take a final bow, dear fellow adventurers, carry this empowering journey in your hearts, and may your health adventure continue to sparkle like a constellation of self-care, love, and empowerment!

About the Author

Meet Dr. Anjum, a mother, entrepreneur, Healthtech and public health expert. She is the visionary founder of EveCare, with a vision to be at the forefront of women's healthcare, providing innovative and knowledge driven tech solutions, thereby empowering women at every stage of life to prioritize their health and well-being.

Dr. Anjum, has made significant contributions during her work with the NHA-Government of India for ABPM-JAY. As Vice President at IHX, she has revolutionized Indian healthcare through data and technology, aiming to improve healthcare delivery for all.

Beyond her entrepreneurial venture, Dr. Anjum's accomplishments include successfully leading the implementation of MediBuddy during her tenure at MediAssist. Her educational journey is equally impressive, with a master's in healthcare management and a bachelor's in homeopathic medicine & Surgery, completed in 2011 and 2005, respectively. Recognized as the "Inspiring Leader of the Year 2018" at the Third Future Women Leader Summit and Awards by Transformance.

Dr. Anjum's dedication to empowering women and transforming healthcare has positioned her as a visionary leader, leaving a lasting impact on the lives of countless individuals.

She's on a mission to improve women's health and education globally.